ROLFING FOR STRUCTURAL HEALTH

Comprehensive Techniques For Postural Alignment, Pain Relief, And Enhanced Mobility

DR. MELISSA STOTLER

Disclaimer:

The data in this book, is solely meant to be informative and instructional.

This book is not intended to replace expert medical advice, diagnosis, or care. No medical, health, or other professional services are offered by the author, publisher, or any affiliated parties

Individual outcomes may differ in the practice of these therapies, which entail a variety of approaches and methodologies.

A one-on-one session with a trained or certified healthcare professional is still preferable. It is best to consult a trained healthcare provider before making any decisions regarding your health.

The author of this book is not affiliated with any specific website, product, or organization related to any of these therapies.

All reasonable measures have been taken by the author and publisher to guarantee the authenticity and dependability of the material contained in this book.

Contents

ABOUT THIS BOOK

"Rolfing for Structural Health" delves deeply into the transformative potential of Rolfing, offering a comprehensive exploration of this unique approach to bodywork. By tracing its historical roots from its origins through its evolution and modern adaptations, the book provides a solid foundation for understanding how Rolfing has developed into a powerful tool for structural health. It highlights the contributions of key figures and the progressive techniques that have shaped Rolfing's current practices.

At the heart of the book are the core principles of Rolfing, including the ten-series approach, the integration of body alignment, and the focus on the fascial system. The role of gravity and the balancing of structural and functional aspects are meticulously examined, providing readers with a clear understanding of the underlying philosophy that drives Rolfing.

The book takes a practical approach by detailing the Rolfing process, from initial assessment to the techniques used in each session. It guides readers through the step-by-step progression of sessions, offering insights into how effectiveness and results are measured. This practical perspective is complemented by a thorough discussion of the benefits of Rolfing, which range from improved posture and flexibility to relief from chronic pain and enhanced overall well-being.

Special attention is given to Rolfing's application for specific conditions, including back pain, joint issues, and muscle tension. The book also offers guidance on choosing a qualified Rolf practitioner, preparing for sessions, and addressing common concerns, ensuring readers are well-informed and prepared for their Rolfing journey.

With a section dedicated to frequently asked questions, readers will gain clarity on how Rolfing differs from other therapies, what to expect if sessions are missed, and the long-term benefits of this practice. This book is designed to elevate your understanding and appreciation of Rolfing, equipping you with the knowledge to harness its full potential for structural health.

History and Evolution of Rolfing

Origins of Rolfing

Rolfing, also known as Structural Integration, began in the mid-20th century with the pioneering work of Ida Rolf, an American biochemist. Dr. Rolf developed this method based on her understanding of connective tissue (fascia) and its role in the body's structural integrity. Her initial studies and practices focused on how the alignment of the body's structure affects overall health and well-being. Drawing from her background in biomechanics and her studies with other influential figures in the field of physical therapy, Rolf crafted a system that emphasized realigning and balancing the body's structure to improve posture and reduce pain.

Development Through the Years

After its inception, Rolfing gained traction in the 1970s and 1980s as more practitioners adopted and adapted her techniques. The method was initially introduced to the public through workshops and training programs that Dr. Rolf herself conducted. Over the years, as Rolfing's popularity grew, various practitioners began to refine and expand upon the original techniques. This period saw the emergence of different schools of thought within Rolfing, each contributing to the method's evolution. Practitioners started integrating concepts from other therapeutic disciplines, such as osteopathy and massage therapy, to enhance and diversify the approach.

Key Figures and Contributors

Several key figures have played crucial roles in the evolution of Rolfing. Besides Ida Rolf, notable contributors include her early students and the practitioners who helped to disseminate her teachings. Dr. Rolf's students, such as Peter Melchior and Franklin Sills, were instrumental in expanding the practice beyond its original scope. These individuals not only helped to train new practitioners but also contributed to the development of new techniques and theories within the Rolfing community. Their collective efforts have been vital in establishing Rolfing as a respected method of bodywork and structural integration.

Evolution of Techniques and Methods

Rolfing has undergone significant changes since its inception. Early Rolfing techniques primarily focused on manipulating the fascia to release tension and improve alignment. As the practice evolved, practitioners began incorporating more refined techniques and approaches. This included the development of systematic approaches to bodywork that aimed to address specific patterns of tension and imbalance. Additionally, the integration of other therapeutic modalities, such as craniosacral therapy and movement education, has enriched the Rolfing practice, allowing practitioners to address a broader range of issues and individual needs.

Modern Adaptations and Practices

In recent years, Rolfing has continued to evolve with the integration of modern practices and technological advancements. Contemporary Rolfing practitioners often blend traditional techniques with innovations from fields like functional movement and sports therapy. The emphasis has shifted toward a more holistic approach that considers the interplay between physical, emotional, and environmental factors in structural health. Modern Rolfing practices frequently incorporate assessments using advanced tools and methods to tailor treatments more precisely to individual needs. This ongoing adaptation ensures that Rolfing remains relevant and effective in addressing the diverse needs of today's clients.

CHAPTER ONE

CORE PRINCIPLES OF ROLFING

Rolfing, a form of structural integration, is based on a few core principles that guide its approach to improving physical alignment and function.

These principles revolve around understanding the body's structure, its alignment, and how various systems interact. Let's delve into each of these principles to grasp the fundamentals of Rolfing.

The Ten Series Approach

The Ten Series is a foundational concept in Rolfing that involves a systematic approach to bodywork.

This series consists of ten sessions, each designed to address specific aspects of the body's structure. The approach begins with assessing and improving overall body alignment and progressively targets deeper structural issues.

Each session in the Ten Series focuses on different areas, from the superficial layers of the body to the deeper, more intricate fascial connections.

The first few sessions typically work on broadening and aligning the body, while the later sessions delve into more specialized areas, such as the pelvic and thoracic regions.

This progressive, step-by-step approach ensures a thorough and effective realignment, helping to release long-standing tensions and improve overall body function.

Integrating Body Alignment

Body alignment is a central focus in Rolfing. It involves realigning the body's structural components—bones, muscles, and connective tissues—to achieve a more balanced and functional posture.

When the body is misaligned, it can lead to discomfort, pain, and inefficient movement patterns.

Rolfing aims to correct these misalignments by re-educating the body to maintain proper alignment.

This is done through a combination of hands-on techniques and guided movements. The goal is to achieve a more natural and efficient alignment, which can enhance movement, reduce pain, and improve overall well-being.

Working With The Fascial System

The fascial system plays a crucial role in Rolfing. Fascia is the connective tissue that surrounds and supports muscles, bones, and organs.

It forms a continuous network throughout the body and significantly influences how we move and feel.

Rolfing techniques involve working with this fascial system to release restrictions and improve flexibility.

By applying pressure and manipulating the fascia, Rolfing practitioners help to break up adhesions and improve the body's range of motion.

This not only helps in alleviating pain but also supports better movement patterns and structural balance.

The Role Of Gravity In Rolfing

Gravity is an important consideration in Rolfing. It affects how we carry our weight and how our bodies respond to gravitational forces. Misalignment and poor posture can lead to inefficient use of gravity, resulting in strain and discomfort.

Rolfing addresses the role of gravity by helping the body find a more balanced and efficient posture.

By realigning the body and improving its relationship with gravity, Rolfing helps to reduce the stress placed on various structures and supports a more natural and effortless movement.

This can lead to improved posture, reduced strain, and a more harmonious interaction with gravitational forces.

Balancing Structural And Functional Aspects

In Rolfing, balancing structural and functional aspects is key to achieving long-term improvements. Structural work focuses on aligning and balancing the body's physical components, while functional work addresses how these components work together during movement.

Rolfing seeks to harmonize these aspects by not only correcting physical misalignments but also enhancing functional movement patterns. This approach ensures that the body is not only properly aligned but also able to move efficiently and effectively. By addressing both structural and functional elements, Rolfing aims to provide a comprehensive solution to discomfort and movement limitations.

CHAPTER TWO

THE ROLFING PROCESS

Initial Assessment And Evaluation

The journey with Rolfing begins with a comprehensive assessment to understand your body's current state and identify areas that may need attention. During this initial evaluation, your Rolfer will conduct a thorough physical examination, assessing your posture, movement patterns, and any specific discomfort or pain you may be experiencing. This evaluation helps in creating a tailored plan to address your unique needs.

The Rolfer will ask about your medical history, lifestyle, and any previous injuries to gain a complete picture of your body's condition. They may also use various tools, such as visual assessments and movement tests, to gauge your structural alignment and flexibility. This foundational assessment is crucial for setting goals and determining the most effective approach for your Rolfing sessions.

Step-By-Step Guide To A Typical Session

A typical Rolfing session is designed to be both thorough and focused. It generally begins with a discussion between you and your Rolfer about any changes or observations since your last session. This allows for any necessary adjustments to the treatment plan.

The session itself usually starts with some form of gentle warming up or stretching to prepare your body. The Rolfer then employs a variety of hands-on techniques to manipulate and release tension in your fascia. This may involve deep tissue work, gentle stretching, and other specialized movements aimed at improving alignment and flexibility.

Throughout the session, your Rolfer will communicate with you, checking in on your comfort levels and adjusting their approach as needed. The goal is to work with your body's natural responses to gradually improve its structure and function. Each session typically lasts between 60 to 90 minutes, depending on the areas being addressed and your individual needs.

Techniques Used In Rolfing

Rolfing employs a range of techniques to target the fascia, the connective tissue that surrounds muscles and organs. One common technique is deep tissue manipulation, where the Rolfer uses their fingers, elbows, or other tools to apply pressure and release tightness in the fascia. This can help to realign the body's structure and improve movement.

Another technique is myofascial release, which involves applying gentle, sustained pressure to the fascia to relieve tension and restore flexibility. The Rolfer may also use stretching techniques to enhance the length and elasticity of the fascia, contributing to improved posture and movement.

Rolfing may also include movement re-education, where the Rolfer guides you through specific exercises and stretches designed to help you integrate the changes achieved during the session into your daily activities. These techniques are tailored to address your individual needs and goals, ensuring a personalized approach to improving your structural health.

Progression Of Sessions

The progression of Rolfing sessions typically follows a structured approach, beginning with a series of foundational sessions aimed at addressing major structural imbalances. Initially, sessions may focus on releasing deep-seated tension and aligning the body's core structures.

As you progress, the focus may shift towards more specific areas or issues, such as improving mobility in certain

joints or enhancing overall posture. The number of sessions required can vary based on individual needs and goals, but a common approach involves a series of 10 to 12 sessions, each building upon the previous ones.

Throughout the process, your Rolfer will continually assess your progress and adjust the treatment plan as necessary. This ensures that the sessions remain effective and aligned with your evolving needs. The progression is designed to be gradual and supportive, allowing your body to adapt and integrate the changes over time.

Measuring Effectiveness And Results

Measuring the effectiveness of Rolfing involves both subjective and objective assessments. Subjectively, you may notice improvements in how you feel, such as reduced pain, increased flexibility, and improved posture.

Your Rolfer will regularly check in with you to discuss any changes in symptoms or overall well-being.

Objectively, effectiveness can be measured through physical assessments, such as changes in range of motion, posture, and alignment.

Your Rolfer may use tools like postural analysis or movement tests to track progress and evaluate the results of the sessions.

The overall effectiveness of Rolfing is often seen in the long-term benefits, such as enhanced movement patterns, better posture, and a reduction in chronic pain or tension.

The goal is to achieve lasting improvements in your structural health, contributing to a more balanced and functional body.

CHAPTER THREE

BENEFITS OF ROLFING

Improved Posture And Alignment

Rolfing is renowned for its ability to enhance posture and alignment. This technique targets the connective tissues, known as fascia, to release tension and restore the body's natural alignment.

By working through the layers of fascia, Rolfing helps to correct imbalances that affect posture.

As a result, you may notice a more upright stance and balanced alignment, which can reduce strain on muscles and joints.

Improved posture not only alleviates physical discomfort but also boosts confidence and presence.

Enhanced Movement And Flexibility

One of the most celebrated benefits of Rolfing is its impact on movement and flexibility. The process involves deep tissue manipulation that helps to release restrictions in the fascia. This release allows for a greater range of motion and smoother movement.

As your body becomes more flexible, everyday activities become easier, and athletic performance can improve. Whether you're a dancer, athlete, or simply someone looking to move more comfortably, Rolfing can help you achieve greater physical freedom and ease.

Relief From Chronic Pain

Chronic pain can significantly impact the quality of life, but Rolfing offers a promising approach to relief. By addressing the underlying fascial restrictions and imbalances, Rolfing targets the root causes of pain rather than just masking symptoms. This holistic approach can lead to significant reductions in discomfort and improvements in overall functionality. Many individuals report a decrease in pain levels and an enhanced ability to engage in activities without being hindered by persistent discomfort.

Better Body Awareness

Rolfing promotes a heightened sense of body awareness, which is crucial for overall health and well-being.

Through the process, you develop a deeper understanding of how your body moves and feels.

This increased awareness helps you recognize and correct habitual patterns that may contribute to tension or pain. As you become more in tune with your body, you can make more informed decisions about posture, movement, and self-care, leading to a more harmonious and balanced physical experience.

Increased Overall Well-Being

The benefits of Rolfing extend beyond physical improvements to enhance overall well-being. By addressing structural imbalances and releasing tension, Rolfing contributes to a sense of relaxation and mental clarity. The process can help alleviate stress, improve sleep, and boost mood, leading to a more positive outlook on life. As physical discomfort diminishes and body awareness increases, many individuals find that their overall quality of life improves, making Rolfing a valuable practice for holistic health.

CHAPTER FOUR

ROLFING FOR SPECIFIC CONDITIONS

Managing Back Pain

Rolfing can be an effective approach for managing back pain by addressing the underlying structural imbalances.

The therapy focuses on the connective tissue, known as fascia, which plays a crucial role in supporting the spine and surrounding muscles. During a Rolfing session for back pain, the practitioner uses deep tissue manipulation to release tension and realign the fascia.

This process helps to improve posture, reduce muscle stiffness, and restore proper alignment to the spine. By addressing these issues, Rolfing can relieve pressure on nerves and reduce discomfort, providing lasting relief from chronic back pain.

In addition to hands-on techniques, Rolfing incorporates movement education to help clients develop better body awareness and alignment.

This helps individuals learn how to move more efficiently, reducing strain on the back and preventing future pain. Regular Rolfing sessions can contribute to long-term improvements in spinal health and overall comfort.

Addressing Joint Issues

Rolfing can be beneficial for individuals dealing with joint issues by improving the overall alignment and function of the body. Joints rely on the surrounding fascia and muscles to maintain proper movement and stability.

When these structures are misaligned or tense, it can lead to joint pain and dysfunction. Through targeted Rolfing techniques, practitioners work to release tightness in the fascia and restore balance to the affected areas.

For joint issues, Rolfing often includes techniques that focus on improving joint mobility and reducing restrictions in the surrounding tissues.

By enhancing the flexibility and alignment of the fascia, Rolfing can help reduce inflammation and pain in the joints.

This approach also aids in improving overall movement patterns, which can alleviate stress on the joints and support better joint health over time.

Alleviating Muscle Tension

Muscle tension can be a significant source of discomfort and pain, and Rolfing offers a practical approach to alleviating this tension. The therapy targets the fascia, which surrounds and connects the muscles throughout the body. By applying deep, sustained pressure to specific areas, Rolfing helps to release built-up tension and restore normal muscle function.

In a typical session, the Rolfing practitioner uses a combination of techniques to address areas of tightness and restriction. This might include deep tissue work, myofascial release, and stretching. The goal is to help the muscles relax, improve blood flow, and enhance overall muscle elasticity. As a result, clients often experience reduced pain, increased flexibility, and improved range of motion.

Improving Athletic Performance

Rolfing can play a key role in enhancing athletic performance by optimizing the body's structural alignment and function. Athletes often experience imbalances and restrictions in their fascia that can impact their performance and increase the risk of injury. Rolfing addresses these issues by focusing on the body's connective tissues and improving overall alignment.

During Rolfing sessions, athletes benefit from improved posture, better movement efficiency, and enhanced flexibility.

By releasing restrictions in the fascia and aligning the body, Rolfing helps athletes move more freely and efficiently. This can lead to increased strength, endurance, and agility. Additionally, Rolfing can aid in injury prevention by addressing underlying imbalances that may contribute to strain or overuse injuries.

Supporting Recovery From Injuries

Rolfing can be a valuable tool for supporting recovery from injuries by facilitating the body's natural healing processes.

After an injury, the body often develops compensatory patterns and tightness in the fascia, which can hinder recovery and contribute to ongoing discomfort. Rolfing helps to address these issues by focusing on the release of restrictions and the restoration of proper alignment.

Through targeted techniques, Rolfing aids in reducing pain, improving mobility, and promoting better overall function.

The therapy also supports the healing of soft tissues by enhancing blood flow and reducing scar tissue formation.

As clients progress through their recovery, Rolfing can help restore normal movement patterns and prevent future complications, contributing to a more effective and efficient healing process.

CHAPTER FIVE

CHOOSING A ROLF PRACTITIONER

Qualifications And Certifications

When choosing a Rolf practitioner, it's essential to consider their qualifications and certifications. Rolfing, or Structural Integration, is a specialized form of bodywork that requires in-depth training and expertise. Practitioners typically undergo extensive education in anatomy, physiology, and Rolfing techniques. Look for practitioners who are certified by recognized organizations such as the Rolf Institute of Structural Integration or the Guild for Structural Integration. Certification ensures that the practitioner has completed a rigorous training program and adheres to professional standards. Additionally, check for any ongoing education or specialized training that the practitioner might have, as this indicates a commitment to staying updated with the latest techniques and practices in Rolfing.

What To Look For In A Practitioner

Finding the right Rolf practitioner involves more than just checking credentials. Consider the practitioner's experience and areas of specialization. An experienced practitioner is likely to have a deeper understanding of complex structural issues and a more refined touch. Assess their approach to Rolfing—do they focus on specific goals or work with a broad range of clients? Look for reviews or testimonials from past clients to get a sense of their effectiveness and how they interact with clients. It's also important to find someone who communicates clearly and seems genuinely interested in understanding your needs. A practitioner who listens to your concerns and adapts their approach to suit your requirements is more likely to provide a successful Rolfing experience.

Questions To Ask During A Consultation

During your initial consultation with a Rolf practitioner, ask questions to gauge their suitability for your needs. Start by inquiring about their training and certification to ensure they have the necessary qualifications.

Ask about their experience with conditions similar to yours and the types of clients they usually work with.

It's also helpful to discuss their approach to Rolfing—how do they plan to address your specific issues, and what techniques will they use? Clarify the duration and frequency of sessions, as well as the expected outcomes and how they measure progress.

Finally, discuss the cost of sessions and whether they offer any package deals or sliding scale fees. These questions will help you determine if the practitioner's approach aligns with your goals and if their services fit within your budget.

Understanding Different Practitioner Styles

Rolfing practitioners often have different styles and approaches, which can significantly impact your experience. Some practitioners might focus on deep tissue work to address specific structural issues, while others might adopt a more gentle approach aimed at overall balance and alignment. Understanding these styles can help you choose a practitioner whose methods resonate with your needs. For instance, if you prefer a hands-on approach that targets deep-seated tension, look for a practitioner known

CHAPTER SIX

PREPARING FOR YOUR ROLFING SESSIONS

Setting Goals And Expectations

Before beginning your Rolfing sessions, it's crucial to define your goals and set clear expectations. Start by reflecting on what you hope to achieve from the process. Are you seeking relief from chronic pain, improving your posture, or enhancing overall body alignment? Write down your specific goals and discuss them with your Rolfing practitioner. This helps ensure that both you and your practitioner are on the same page and can tailor the sessions to meet your needs effectively.

Additionally, understanding that Rolfing is a gradual process can help set realistic expectations. Results may not be immediate, and improvement often occurs over a series of sessions. Be patient and open to the journey, and remember that progress is often incremental.

Preparing Mentally And Physically

Preparing for Rolfing involves both mental and physical readiness. Mentally, approach the sessions with an open mind and a willingness to engage in the process. Rolfing can involve exploring areas of tension and discomfort, and being mentally prepared can make this experience more manageable. Practice relaxation techniques such as deep breathing or mindfulness to help calm your mind before each session.

Physically, it's important to be in a comfortable state. Ensure that you are well-hydrated, as drinking plenty of water helps keep your tissues hydrated and responsive to the Rolfing techniques. Avoid strenuous exercise or heavy meals immediately before your session, as this can make you feel uncomfortable during the process.

What To Wear And Bring

For your Rolfing sessions, wear loose, comfortable clothing that allows for easy movement. Avoid wearing restrictive or tight-fitting clothes, as they can interfere with the practitioner's ability to assess and work on your body effectively. Many practitioners recommend wearing athletic wear or clothing that is breathable and flexible.

Bring a water bottle to stay hydrated, and consider bringing a small towel or blanket for added comfort if needed. It's also helpful to bring any personal items you might need, such as a change of clothes or a snack for after the session.

Being prepared with these essentials helps you stay comfortable and focused during your Rolfing experience.

Managing Discomfort Or Sensitivity

It's common to experience some discomfort or sensitivity during and after Rolfing sessions. This is often a sign that your body is releasing tension and adjusting to the changes. Communicate openly with your practitioner about any discomfort you experience. They can adjust their techniques or offer modifications to better suit your comfort level.

To manage post-session discomfort, consider gentle stretching or applying a warm compress to areas that feel sore.

Rest and take it easy for the remainder of the day, allowing your body to recover and integrate the work done during the session. Keeping a journal to track your experiences and any changes you notice can also be useful for understanding how your body is responding.

Creating A Supportive Environment

Creating a supportive environment for your Rolfing sessions helps enhance the overall experience. Choose a quiet, relaxing space for your sessions, free from distractions and interruptions.

If your sessions are held at a practitioner's office, ensure that it is a calm and inviting space that promotes relaxation.

At home, create a post-session environment that supports your body's recovery. Set aside time to rest and engage in activities that help you relax and unwind, such as gentle stretching, reading, or taking a warm bath. Having a supportive environment both during and after your sessions helps maximize the benefits of Rolfing and contributes to a more positive and effective experience.

CHAPTER SEVEN

COMMON CONCERNS AND HOW TO ADDRESS THEM

Pain Or Discomfort During Sessions

It's normal to experience some level of discomfort during Rolfing sessions, especially if your body is adjusting to new patterns of movement and alignment. This discomfort often stems from the deep work involved in Rolfing, which targets the fascia—the connective tissue that surrounds muscles and organs. The intensity can vary based on your body's current state and how accustomed it is to this type of manipulation.

To manage discomfort, communicate openly with your Rolfer about any pain you experience. They can adjust their techniques or pressure to suit your comfort level. It's also helpful to practice deep breathing and relaxation techniques during sessions to ease tension. Remember, while some discomfort is expected, it should not be unbearable or persistent. If you experience severe pain, it's crucial to let your Rolfer know immediately so they can make the necessary adjustments.

Expectations Vs. Reality

Many people come to Rolfing with high expectations of immediate relief or dramatic changes. While some individuals might experience noticeable improvements after just a few sessions, Rolfing is generally a process that unfolds over time. The changes in posture, alignment, and movement can be gradual, and the effects might not be immediately visible.

It's important to set realistic goals and understand that Rolfing works to reorganize and release patterns that have developed over the years. This can take time and requires patience. Work with your Rolfer to establish clear goals and a timeline for your treatment. Keeping a journal of your progress and any changes you notice can help manage expectations and provide motivation throughout your Rolfing journey.

Frequency And Duration Of Sessions

The frequency and duration of Rolfing sessions can vary depending on individual needs and goals. Typically, clients start with a series of 10 sessions, each lasting between 60 to 90 minutes. These sessions are usually spaced one to two weeks apart to allow your body time to integrate the changes made during each session.

Your Rolfer will tailor the schedule based on your specific needs and how your body responds to the work.

It's important to attend sessions regularly, especially at the beginning, to achieve the best results.

After the initial series, some clients may choose to continue with periodic maintenance sessions to reinforce the benefits and address any new issues that arise.

Integrating Rolfing With Other Therapies

Rolfing can be effectively integrated with other therapies and treatments. Many people find that combining Rolfing with physical therapy, chiropractic care, or massage therapy enhances their overall results.

The key is to coordinate with your healthcare providers to ensure that the therapies complement each other and do not interfere with your Rolfing progress.

Discuss any other treatments you're receiving with your Rolfer. They can help you determine the best approach and timing for combining therapies. It's often helpful to stagger sessions or focus on different aspects of your health with each therapy to avoid overwhelming your body.

Cost And Insurance Considerations

The cost of Rolfing can vary based on location, practitioner experience, and session length. Typically, each session ranges from $100 to $200, and most practitioners recommend a series of 10 sessions. It's wise to inquire about the total cost upfront and check if any package deals are available.

Insurance coverage for Rolfing can be limited or non-existent, as it is often considered an alternative therapy.

However, some flexible spending accounts (FSAs) or health savings accounts (HSAs) may cover Rolfing's expenses. Check with your insurance provider to see if you have any coverage options or reimbursement possibilities. If not, discussing payment plans or sliding scale fees with your Rolfer can help manage costs.

By addressing these common concerns, you can approach Rolfing with greater confidence and clarity, making the experience more effective and enjoyable.

CHAPTER EIGHT

FAQS ABOUT ROLFING

How Does Rolfing Differ From Massage Therapy?

Rolfing and massage therapy both focus on the body's soft tissues, but they approach treatment with different goals and techniques. Massage therapy typically targets muscle relaxation and alleviates tension through various strokes and manipulations. It often provides immediate relief and promotes relaxation, making it a popular choice for stress management.

Rolfing, or Rolfing Structural Integration, is a more comprehensive approach. It aims to align and balance the body's structure by working on the connective tissue, known as fascia, which surrounds and supports muscles and organs.

Rolfing sessions are usually longer and more in-depth, focusing on the body's overall alignment and function rather than just muscle relaxation. This method seeks to address postural imbalances, improve movement efficiency, and create lasting changes in the body's structure.

In essence, while massage therapy is often used for relaxation and immediate muscle relief, Rolfing is designed to address structural imbalances and long-term physical changes by working on the body's deeper connective tissues.

What Should I Do If I Miss A Session?

Missing a Rolfing session can impact the continuity and effectiveness of your treatment plan. If you miss a session, it's essential to contact your Rolfing practitioner as soon as possible to reschedule. Many practitioners offer flexible scheduling options to accommodate missed appointments.

To minimize the effects of missing a session, try to maintain any recommended self-care practices or exercises provided by your Rolfing practitioner. These exercises are designed to support your progress and can help maintain the benefits achieved during previous sessions. It's also a good idea to communicate openly with your practitioner about any issues or challenges you are facing, as they can guide how to stay on track with your treatment plan.

How Long Will It Take To See Results?

The time it takes to see results from Rolfing can vary depending on several factors, including the individual's condition, the goals of the treatment, and the frequency of sessions.

Generally, clients may start to notice some improvements after a few sessions. These initial changes might include increased ease of movement, reduced discomfort, and better body awareness.

Rolfing is often conducted in a series of sessions, typically ranging from 10 to 12, designed to progressively address different aspects of the body's structure.

Significant and lasting changes in posture, movement patterns, and overall comfort may take more time, often several weeks or months.

It's important to maintain open communication with your Rolfing practitioner and adhere to any recommended home practices to support the process and achieve the best results.

Can Rolfing Help With Chronic Conditions?

Yes, Rolfing can be beneficial for managing and potentially improving various chronic conditions. By focusing on the body's connective tissues and overall alignment, Rolfing aims to address structural imbalances that may contribute to chronic pain, tension, and dysfunction. Conditions such as chronic back pain, repetitive strain injuries, and postural issues often benefit from Rolfing's approach.

While Rolfing may help alleviate symptoms and improve function, it's important to approach it as a complementary therapy. Combining Rolfing with other treatments and therapies, as well as maintaining a healthy lifestyle, can enhance overall outcomes. Always consult with your healthcare provider to ensure that Rolfing is appropriate for your specific condition and to develop a comprehensive treatment plan.

What Are The Long-Term Benefits Of Rolfing?

Rolfing offers several long-term benefits that extend beyond immediate relief of discomfort. One of the primary advantages is improved body alignment and posture. By addressing structural imbalances and enhancing the body's natural alignment, Rolfing can lead to better movement efficiency, reduced strain on muscles and joints, and a more balanced and functional body.

Other long-term benefits include increased flexibility and range of motion, which can enhance physical performance and prevent injuries. Many individuals also experience improved body awareness, which helps in maintaining good posture and ergonomic practices in daily activities. Additionally, by addressing the root causes of chronic discomfort or tension, Rolfing can contribute to long-term relief and overall well-being.

By maintaining regular sessions and incorporating any self-care practices recommended by your Rolfing practitioner, you can sustain and build upon these benefits for lasting improvements in your structural health.